Barbara O'Neill Herbal Remedies Complete Collection

A Comprehensive Guide to Health and Healing for Wellness, Vitality, and Holistic Living.

Diala Samuel

Barbara O'Neill Herbal Remedies

This book is a comprehensive guide to understanding and utilizing the herbal remedies advocated by Barbara O'Neill, offering insights into natural healing methods and their applications. The information contained herein is intended for educational purposes and is not a substitute for professional medical advice, diagnosis, or treatment.

Barbara O'Neill Herbal Remedies

Table of Contents

Barbara O'Neill Herbal Remedies

Barbara O'Neill Herbal Remedies

Barbara O'Neill Herbal Remedies

Barbara O'Neill Herbal Remedies

Barbara O'Neill Herbal Remedies

Barbara O'Neill Herbal Remedies

Barbara O'Neill Herbal Remedies

Barbara O'Neill Herbal Remedies

INTRODUCTION

Barbara O'Neill is a renowned herbalist and holistic health educator whose work has significantly contributed to the field of natural medicine. With a deep-seated passion for herbal healing and a commitment to empowering individuals with knowledge about plant-based remedies, Barbara has become a respected voice in the world of herbalism.

Her approach combines traditional wisdom with modern scientific understanding, offering a comprehensive and practical perspective on using herbs for health and well-being. Barbara's teachings emphasize the importance of a holistic approach to health—one that recognizes the interconnectedness of the body, mind, and spirit.

In this collection, "Barbara O'Neill Herbal Remedies Complete Collection," A Comprehensive Guide to Health and Healing" for your Wellness, Vitality, and Holistic Living, you will find a wealth of information drawn from her extensive experience and expertise. This book is designed to guide you through the fundamentals of herbal medicine, provide practical remedies for common ailments, and offer insights into integrating herbal practices into your daily life.

Barbara O'Neill Herbal Remedies

What You Can Expect:

- **Foundational Knowledge**: Gain a thorough understanding of herbal medicine, including its history, scientific basis, and preparation methods. Barbara's clear and accessible explanations will help you build a solid foundation in herbal practices.

- **Practical Remedies**: Explore targeted herbal solutions for a variety of common health conditions. Barbara's remedies are based on her extensive experience and knowledge, providing effective, natural alternatives for managing and improving your health.

- **Holistic Lifestyle Integration**: Learn how to incorporate herbal remedies into your daily life, from creating an herbal medicine cabinet to growing your own herbs. Barbara's practical advice will help you embrace a holistic lifestyle that supports overall well-being.

- **Inspiration and Empowerment**: Barbara's work is not just about using herbs; it's about empowering you to take charge of your health and well-being. Her approach encourages self-discovery, experimentation, and a deeper connection with nature.

Barbara O'Neill Herbal Remedies

Whether you are new to herbal medicine or looking to expand your knowledge, Barbara O'Neill's insights and remedies offer a valuable resource for enhancing your health and living a more natural, balanced life. This book serves as a comprehensive guide, drawing on Barbara's wisdom and experience to support your journey into the world of herbal healing.

In an era dominated by modern medicine and pharmaceuticals, the allure of herbal remedies persists as a timeless testament to humanity's profound relationship with nature. For millennia, civilizations across the globe have relied on the healing properties of plants to alleviate ailments, soothe discomforts, and promote overall well-being.

In this book, we embark on a journey through the world of herbal remedies, exploring their origins, applications, and scientific basis. From ancient herbalists who cultivated extensive knowledge through trial and observation to contemporary scientists unraveling the bioactive compounds within plants, the evolution of herbal medicine reflects both the continuity of tradition and the innovation of modern research.

Barbara O'Neill's Herbal remedies encompass a diverse array of preparations, from teas and tinctures to poultices and essential oils, each crafted to harness the therapeutic potential of botanical sources. Whether addressing common colds, digestive issues, stress, or

Barbara O'Neill Herbal Remedies

chronic conditions, herbs offer a holistic approach that complements conventional medical treatments.

Moreover, understanding herbal remedies extends beyond their medicinal applications. It invites us to reconnect with the natural world, to appreciate the intricate ecosystems that sustain life, and to recognize the profound wisdom encoded in plants. Each herb tells a story of adaptation, resilience, and adaptation—a narrative woven into the fabric of human history.

As we delve into the pages ahead, we invite you to explore the rich tapestry of herbal remedies—a tapestry that merges ancient wisdom with modern science, offering pathways to health and wellness that are as relevant today as they were centuries ago. Together, let us uncover the secrets of nature's pharmacy and discover the transformative power of herbal medicine.

Barbara O'Neill Herbal Remedies

CHAPTER ONE

HISTORY AND EVOLUTION

Throughout history, herbal remedies have been integral to human healing practices across cultures and continents. The roots of herbal medicine can be traced back thousands of years to ancient civilizations such as the Egyptians, Greeks, Chinese, and Indigenous peoples around the world. These early societies relied on the abundant plant life around them to treat ailments and maintain health.

Ancient Practices:

The history of herbal medicine parallels that of human civilization. Early humans discovered that certain plants had the power to heal wounds, cure illnesses, and enhance overall well-being. Ancient texts from civilizations such as Egypt, China, and India provide detailed records of medicinal plants and their uses. In ancient Egypt, for instance, herbs like garlic and juniper were used to treat various ailments. Traditional Chinese Medicine (TCM) boasts a long history, with texts like the "Shennong Ben Cao Jing" documenting the medicinal properties of hundreds of herbs. Similarly, Ayurveda, the traditional medicine of India, has utilized herbs such as turmeric and ashwagandha for thousands of years.

Barbara O'Neill Herbal Remedies

Modern Applications:

While modern medicine has made incredible advancements, there is a growing recognition of the value of traditional herbal remedies. Many pharmaceutical drugs are derived from plant compounds, and the integration of herbal medicine into mainstream healthcare is increasing. The World Health Organization (WHO) acknowledges the importance of traditional medicine and promotes its safe and effective use.

Current Trends:

Herbal medicine is still developing today, with numerous traditional uses being validated by modern investigation. There is a growing interest in integrative medicine, which combines conventional medical treatments with complementary therapies like herbal medicine to achieve optimal health outcomes.

Understanding the historical context of herbal remedies provides insight into their enduring popularity and efficacy. As we delve into specific herbs and their applications in this book, we recognize the wisdom of ancient healers while embracing contemporary scientific advancements in herbal medicine.

Barbara O'Neill Herbal Remedies

The Benefits and Risks of Herbal Medicine:

Quality Control: The quality of herbal products can vary widely. It's crucial to source herbs from reputable suppliers to ensure purity and potency.

Potential Side Effects: Like any substance, herbs can cause side effects or allergic reactions in some individuals. Numerous traditional uses of herbal medicine have been confirmed by contemporary research, and the field is continuously evolving.

Lack of Regulation: In many countries, herbal supplements are not regulated as strictly as pharmaceuticals. Variability in product safety and quality may result from this.

Herb-Drug Interactions: Some herbs can interact with prescription medications, affecting their effectiveness or causing adverse effects. It's important to consult with a healthcare provider before combining herbs with medications.

Misinformation: There is a vast amount of information available on herbal remedies, not all of which is accurate or evidence-based. It's important to rely on credible sources and research when considering herbal treatments.

Understanding the benefits and risks of herbal remedies is essential for making informed decisions about their use. Throughout this book, we will explore specific herbs and their applications,

Barbara O'Neill Herbal Remedies

providing guidance on how to incorporate them safely and effectively into your wellness routine.

CHAPTER TWO
THE BASICS OF HERBAL MEDICINE

What Are Herbs?

Herbs are plants used for their medicinal properties, flavor, and fragrance. They can be leaves, flowers, roots, seeds, or bark. Each part of the plant may have different therapeutic effects. For example, the flowers of chamomile are used to make a calming tea, while the roots of valerian are used as a natural sedative.

How Herbs Work in the Body:

Herbs have active ingredients that interact with the body to provide medicinal benefits. These compounds can include alkaloids, flavonoids, tannins, and essential oils, each with specific actions. For instance, alkaloids can have powerful effects on the nervous system, while flavonoids are known for their antioxidant properties. The synergy of these compounds often enhances their healing potential, making whole herbs more effective than isolated compounds in some cases.

CHAPTER THREE

PREPARING HERBAL REMEDIES

Teas and Infusions

Herbal teas and infusions are the simplest and most common ways to use herbs. They involve steeping herbs in hot water to extract their beneficial compounds. Teas are typically made from leaves and flowers, while infusions are stronger preparations that use roots, bark, and seeds.

Tinctures and Extracts

Herbs are soaked in alcohol or vinegar to create concentrated herbal extracts called tinctures. They last a long time and are very powerful. Extracts can also be made using glycerin or water, depending on the desired properties and intended use.

Salves and Ointments

Salves and ointments are topical preparations made by infusing oils with herbs and then thickening the mixture with beeswax or another

Barbara O'Neill Herbal Remedies

base. They are used to treat skin conditions, wounds, and muscle pain. For instance, a calendula salve can soothe irritated skin, while a comfrey ointment can promote wound healing.

Capsules and Tablets

For convenience and precise dosing, herbs can be encapsulated or made into tablets. This method is particularly useful for herbs with strong tastes or those that are difficult to consume in large quantities. Capsules and tablets also allow for standardized dosages, ensuring consistent therapeutic effects.

Barbara O'Neill Herbal Remedies

Chapter 4

Digestive Health

Good digestive health is essential for overall well-being. Herbal remedies offer gentle and effective ways to support and enhance digestive functions. This chapter explores various herbs that can help with common digestive issues, such as indigestion, acid reflux, constipation, and more.

Herbal Teas for Digestion

Herbal teas can be a soothing and effective way to support digestion. Here are a few well-liked herbs with a reputation for helping digestion:

Peppermint (Mentha piperita): Known for its cooling and soothing properties, peppermint tea can help relieve indigestion, bloating, and gas. It relaxes the muscles of the gastrointestinal tract, making it useful for conditions like irritable bowel syndrome (IBS).

Ginger (Zingiber officinale): Ginger is a powerful digestive aid that helps stimulate saliva, bile, and gastric juices. It is particularly effective for nausea, motion sickness, and indigestion. Fresh ginger tea can be made by steeping sliced ginger root in hot water.

Chamomile (Matricaria chamomilla): Chamomile tea is known for

Barbara O'Neill Herbal Remedies

its calming effects, which can help relax the digestive system and reduce symptoms of indigestion, bloating, and gas. It also has anti-inflammatory properties that can soothe the gastrointestinal tract.

Fennel (Foeniculum vulgare): Fennel seeds are known to relieve bloating, gas, and stomach cramps. Fennel tea can be made by crushing the seeds and steeping them in hot water. It is particularly useful for colic in infants and digestive discomfort in adults.

Remedies for Acid Reflux

When stomach acid refluxes back into the esophagus, it can cause heartburn and other symptoms. Herbal remedies can help soothe and prevent this condition:

Licorice Root (Glycyrrhiza glabra): Licorice root can soothe the stomach lining and reduce inflammation. Deglycyrrhizinated licorice (DGL) is preferred for long-term use to avoid potential side effects from glycyrrhizin, such as high blood pressure.

Slippery Elm (Ulmus rubra): Slippery elm bark contains mucilage, which coats and soothes the esophagus and stomach lining. It can help relieve the symptoms of acid reflux and promote healing of irritated tissues.

Aloe Vera (Aloe barbadensis miller): Aloe vera juice can help reduce inflammation and soothe the gastrointestinal tract. It is

Barbara O'Neill Herbal Remedies

important to use aloe vera juice specifically formulated for internal use to avoid potential laxative effects.

Natural Laxatives

Constipation can be uncomfortable and may lead to other health issues if not addressed. Herbal laxatives can provide gentle relief:

Senna (Senna alexandrina): Senna is a potent herbal laxative that stimulates bowel movements. It should be used sparingly and not for extended periods, as it can cause dependency and affect normal bowel function.

Psyllium (Plantago ovata): Psyllium husk is a natural fiber that adds bulk to stools and promotes regular bowel movements. It is gentle on the digestive system and can be used long-term to support healthy digestion.

Cascara Sagrada (Rhamnus purshiana): Cascara sagrada is a mild herbal laxative that stimulates the muscles of the intestines. It is often used for chronic constipation but should be taken in moderation to avoid dependency.

Flaxseed (Linum usitatissimum): Flaxseeds are high in fiber and can help promote regular bowel movements. Additionally, they offer vital fatty acids that promote general wellness. Ground flaxseeds can be added to foods or taken with water.

Barbara O'Neill Herbal Remedies
Chapter 5

Respiratory Health

Maintaining healthy respiratory function is crucial for overall wellness. Herbal remedies can offer natural support for common respiratory issues such as coughs, colds, asthma, and allergies. This chapter delves into various herbs that can help improve respiratory health and relieve related symptoms.

Herbs for Coughs and Colds

Herbal remedies can be highly effective in alleviating symptoms of coughs and colds, providing relief and promoting quicker recovery.

Echinacea (Echinacea purpurea): Echinacea is known for its immune-boosting properties, making it useful in preventing and reducing the duration of colds. It can be consumed as a pill, tincture, or tea.

Elderberry (Sambucus nigra): Elderberry has antiviral properties that can help fight colds and flu. Elderberry syrup or tea can reduce the severity and length of respiratory infections.

Marshmallow Root (Althaea officinalis): Marshmallow root contains mucilage that soothes irritated mucous membranes in the

Barbara O'Neill Herbal Remedies

throat and respiratory tract. It is beneficial for dry coughs and sore throats.

Thyme (Thymus vulgaris): Thyme has antiseptic and expectorant properties that help clear mucus from the respiratory tract. Thyme tea or steam inhalation can relieve congestion and coughing.

Licorice Root (Glycyrrhiza glabra): Licorice root has anti-inflammatory and soothing properties that can help with sore throats and coughs. It also supports the immune system.

Treatments for Asthma

Asthma is a chronic condition characterized by inflammation and narrowing of the airways. Herbal remedies can help manage symptoms and reduce the frequency of asthma attacks.

Turmeric (Curcuma longa): Turmeric contains curcumin, a powerful anti-inflammatory compound that can help reduce airway inflammation. Turmeric can be taken as a supplement, added to food, or made into a tea.

Gingko Biloba (Gingko biloba): Gingko biloba has been shown to improve lung function and reduce asthma symptoms. It works by decreasing inflammation and improving blood flow to the lungs.

Mullein (Verbascum thapsus): Mullein leaves and flowers are used to make teas and tinctures that can soothe the respiratory tract and

Barbara O'Neill Herbal Remedies

help with asthma symptoms. Mullein acts as an expectorant, clearing mucus from the lungs.

Butterbur (Petasites hybridus): Butterbur has been used to treat asthma and allergies due to its anti-inflammatory and antispasmodic properties. It can be taken as a supplement, but it's essential to use a product free of harmful pyrrolizidine alkaloids (PAs).

Remedies for Allergies

Allergies can cause respiratory symptoms such as sneezing, congestion, and runny nose. Herbal remedies can help alleviate these symptoms and support the immune system.

Nettle (Urtica dioica): Nettle is a natural antihistamine that can help reduce allergy symptoms. Nettle tea or capsules can be taken to alleviate sneezing, itching, and congestion.

Butterbur (Petasites hybridus): Butterbur is effective in treating hay fever and other allergic conditions. It works by inhibiting the release of histamines and leukotrienes, which cause allergic reactions.

Quercetin: One flavonoid that is present in a wide variety of fruits and vegetables is quercetin. It has natural antihistamine and anti-inflammatory properties that can help manage allergy symptoms. Quercetin supplements are available for more concentrated doses.

Barbara O'Neill Herbal Remedies

Eyebright (Euphrasia officinalis): Eyebright has traditionally been used to treat eye-related allergy symptoms such as redness and itching. It can be taken as a tea or used as an eye wash.

Barbara O'Neill Herbal Remedies

CHAPTER SIX

IMMUNE SYSTEM SUPPORT

A robust immune system serves as the cornerstone of optimal health. Herbal remedies can provide natural and effective ways to boost immune function, helping the body fend off illnesses and recover more quickly when sickness does occur. This chapter explores various herbs that support the immune system and offers guidance on incorporating them into your daily routine.

Boosting Immunity Naturally

The following herbs are renowned for their immune-boosting properties and can help enhance the body's natural defenses:

Echinacea (Echinacea purpurea): Echinacea is one of the most well-known herbs for immune support. It stimulates the production of white blood cells, enhancing the body's ability to fight infections. You can consume echinacea as a tea, tincture, or supplement.

Elderberry (Sambucus nigra): Elderberry has strong antiviral properties and is particularly effective against the flu. It boosts the

Barbara O'Neill Herbal Remedies

immune system and reduces the duration and severity of colds and flu. Elderberry syrup, gummies, or tea are popular forms of consumption.

Astragalus (Astragalus membranaceus): Astragalus is an adaptogen that strengthens the immune system and increases resistance to stress and disease. It can be consumed in the form of capsules, tinctures, or tea.

Garlic (Allium sativum): Garlic has antimicrobial and immune-enhancing properties. It can be consumed as a supplement or eaten cooked or raw. Garlic helps combat infections and supports overall immune function.

Ganoderma lucidum, or reishi mushrooms: They are well-known for their ability to modulate the immune system. They help regulate the immune system, making it more efficient at fighting infections. Reishi can be taken as a tea, tincture, or in capsule form.

Herbal Antivirals and Antibacterials

Certain herbs have specific antiviral and antibacterial properties that can help the body fight off infections:

Oregano (Origanum vulgare): Oregano oil is a powerful antimicrobial agent that can combat bacterial and viral infections. Because of its high concentration, it needs to be diluted before usage. Oregano can also be used as a dried herb in cooking.

Barbara O'Neill Herbal Remedies

Olive Leaf (Olea europaea): Olive leaf extract has strong antiviral and antibacterial properties. It can help combat infections and support the immune system. Olive leaf is available as a tincture, capsule, or tea.

Andrographis (Andrographis paniculata): Andrographis is known for its potent antiviral and immune-stimulating properties. It is particularly effective against respiratory infections. Andrographis can be taken as a supplement or tincture.

Lemon Balm (Melissa officinalis): Lemon balm has antiviral properties and is effective against viruses like herpes simplex. It also has calming effects that can help reduce stress, which is beneficial for immune function. Lemon balm can be taken as a tea, tincture, or capsule.

Daily Immune Support

Incorporating immune-supportive herbs into your daily routine can help maintain optimal immune function. Here are some practical tips:

Herbal Teas: Drinking herbal teas regularly is an easy and enjoyable way to boost your immune system. Consider blending herbs like echinacea, elderberry, and astragalus for a potent immune-boosting tea.

Tinctures and Extracts: Tinctures and extracts are concentrated forms of herbs that can be added to water, juice, or tea. They are useful for people who have hectic lives.

Supplements: Herbal supplements, such as capsules and tablets, provide a convenient way to ensure consistent dosing of immune-supportive herbs. Seek out premium goods from reliable vendors.

Incorporating Herbs into Meals: Adding immune-boosting herbs like garlic, oregano, and turmeric to your meals can provide daily support. These herbs can enhance the flavor of your dishes while supporting your health.

CHAPTER SEVEN

SKIN AND HAIR CARE

Healthy skin and hair are not only a reflection of beauty but also of overall wellness. Herbal remedies offer natural and effective ways to nourish and protect your skin and hair, treating various conditions

Barbara O'Neill Herbal Remedies

and promoting health from the inside out. This chapter explores various herbs that support skin and hair care, providing recipes and tips for incorporating them into your routine.

Herbal Solutions for Skin Conditions

Skin issues can range from dryness and acne to more severe conditions like eczema and psoriasis. Herbs can provide relief and promote healing for various skin problems.

Calendula (Calendula officinalis): This herb is well-known for its restorative and anti-inflammatory qualities. It is excellent for treating minor cuts, burns, and skin irritations. Calendula-infused oil or cream can soothe and repair damaged skin.

Aloe Vera (Aloe barbadensis miller): Aloe vera gel is well-known for its soothing and moisturizing properties. It is effective for sunburn, acne, and dry skin. Fresh aloe vera gel can be applied directly to the skin or used in homemade skincare products.

Chamomile (Matricaria chamomilla): Chamomile has anti-inflammatory and calming effects, making it ideal for sensitive and irritated skin. Chamomile tea can be used as a facial rinse, or chamomile-infused oil can be applied to the skin.

Lavender (Lavandula angustifolia): Lavender has antiseptic and anti-inflammatory properties. It can help heal acne, minor cuts, and

Barbara O'Neill Herbal Remedies

burns. Lavender essential oil can be diluted with a carrier oil and applied to the skin or added to baths.

Tea Tree (Melaleuca alternifolia): Tea tree oil is a powerful antiseptic and antimicrobial agent. It is particularly effective for acne and fungal infections. Tea tree oil should be diluted before being applied to the skin to prevent irritation.

Natural Hair Care Remedies

Herbs can enhance hair health, promote growth, and treat common issues like dandruff and hair loss.

Rosemary (Rosmarinus officinalis): Rosemary stimulates hair growth, improves circulation to the scalp, and reduces dandruff. Rosemary-infused oil or a rosemary rinse can be used regularly for healthy hair.

Nettle (Urtica dioica): Nettle is rich in vitamins and minerals that strengthen hair and promote growth. Nettle tea can be used as a hair rinse, or nettle extract can be added to shampoos and conditioners.

Horsetail (Equisetum arvense): Horsetail contains silica, which strengthens hair and improves its texture and shine. Horsetail tea can be used as a hair rinse, or horsetail extract can be added to hair care products.

Barbara O'Neill Herbal Remedies

Amla (Phyllanthus emblica): Amla, also known as Indian gooseberry, is used in Ayurvedic medicine to promote hair growth and prevent premature graying. Amla powder can be mixed with water to create a hair mask, or amla oil can be massaged into the scalp.

Bhringraj (Eclipta prostrata): Bhringraj is known as the "king of herbs" for hair growth. It helps prevent hair loss and promotes healthy, thick hair. Bhringraj oil can be used for scalp massages, or bhringraj powder can be added to hair masks.

DIY Herbal Skincare Recipes

Creating your own herbal skincare products allows you to customize treatments for your specific needs. Here are a few simple recipes:

Soothing Calendula Salve

Ingredients: 1 cup calendula-infused oil, 1/4 cup beeswax

Instructions: Melt the beeswax in a double boiler, add the calendula-infused oil, and stir until well combined. Pour into a jar and let cool. Apply to minor cuts, burns, and dry skin.

Aloe Vera and Lavender Face Mist

Ingredients: 1/2 cup distilled water, 1/4 cup aloe vera gel, 10 drops lavender essential oil.

Instructions: Shake well after mixing all contents in a spray

Barbara O'Neill Herbal Remedies

container. Spritz on the face to hydrate and soothe the skin.

Chamomile and Honey Face Mask

Ingredients: 1 tablespoon dried chamomile flowers, 1 tablespoon raw honey, 2 tablespoons hot water.

Instructions: Steep chamomile flowers in hot water for 10 minutes. Strain and mix the chamomile tea with honey to form a paste. Before rinsing off, apply to the face and let it sit for 15 minutes.

DIY Herbal Hair Care Recipes

Enhance your hair care routine with these herbal recipes:

Rosemary Hair Rinse

Ingredients: 1/4cup dried rosemary, 2cups boiling water

Instructions: Steep rosemary in boiling water for 30 minutes, then strain. Use as a final rinse after shampooing to stimulate hair growth and add shine.

Nourishing Nettle Hair Oil

Ingredients: 1/2 cup nettle-infused oil, 10 drops rosemary essential oil

Instructions: Combine oils in a bottle and shake well. Massage into the scalp and hair, leave on for at least 30 minutes, then wash out.

Barbara O'Neill Herbal Remedies

Amla Hair Mask

Ingredients: 2 tablespoons amla powder, 3-4 tablespoons water (or enough to make a paste).

Instructions: Mix amla powder with water to form a thick paste. After applying to the hair and scalp, carefully rinse after 30 minutes.

CHAPTER EIGHT

WOMEN'S HEALTH

Women's health encompasses a wide range of physical and emotional needs, from menstrual and menopausal symptoms to pregnancy and postpartum care. Herbal remedies offer natural, effective solutions to support women at every stage of life. This chapter explores various herbs that can help address common women's health issues and provides practical guidance for their use.

Menstrual and Menopausal Relief

Herbal remedies can provide significant relief from menstrual discomfort and menopausal symptoms, offering a natural alternative to conventional treatments.

Chasteberry (Vitex agnus-castus): Chasteberry is renowned for its ability to balance hormones and alleviate symptoms of PMS, such as mood swings, breast tenderness, and bloating. It can also help regulate menstrual cycles. Chasteberry is typically taken as a tincture or in capsule form.

Black Cohosh (Cimicifuga racemosa): Black cohosh is commonly used to relieve menopausal symptoms, including hot flashes, night

Barbara O'Neill Herbal Remedies

sweats, and mood swings. It can also help with menstrual cramps. Black cohosh is available as a tea, tincture, or capsule.

Dong Quai (Angelica sinensis): Dong quai is often referred to as "female ginseng" for its ability to support menstrual and reproductive health. It can help regulate menstrual cycles, reduce cramps, and ease menopausal symptoms. Dong quai is usually taken as a tea or in capsule form.

Red Raspberry Leaf (Rubus idaeus): Red raspberry leaf is a tonic for the uterus, helping to tone the muscles and alleviate menstrual cramps. It is also beneficial during pregnancy to prepare the uterus for labor. Red raspberry leaf tea is a popular preparation.

Evening Primrose Oil (Oenothera biennis): Evening primrose oil contains gamma-linolenic acid (GLA), which can help alleviate PMS symptoms and support hormonal balance. It is available in capsule form.

Pregnancy and Postpartum Care

Herbs can offer gentle support during pregnancy and the postpartum period, promoting health and well-being for both mother and baby.

Ginger (Zingiber officinale): Ginger is well-known for its ability to alleviate nausea and morning sickness during pregnancy. Fresh ginger tea or ginger capsules can provide relief from these

Barbara O'Neill Herbal Remedies

symptoms.

Nettle (Urtica dioica): Nettle is rich in vitamins and minerals that support overall health during pregnancy. It can help prevent anemia, support healthy kidney function, and provide essential nutrients. Nettle tea is a gentle and effective way to consume this herb.

Fenugreek (Trigonella foenum-graecum): Fenugreek is often used to support milk production in breastfeeding mothers. Fenugreek seeds can be taken as a tea or in capsule form to help increase milk supply.

Shatavari (Asparagus racemosus): Shatavari is an Ayurvedic herb that supports reproductive health and lactation. It helps balance hormones, increase milk production, and support the body's recovery after childbirth. Shatavari is available as a tincture, powder, or capsule.

Chamomile (Matricaria chamomilla): Chamomile is soothing and calming, making it helpful for promoting relaxation and reducing anxiety during pregnancy and the postpartum period. Chamomile tea is a safe and effective way to enjoy its benefits.

Herbal Support for Specific Conditions

Certain herbs can be particularly beneficial for addressing specific women's health conditions.

Barbara O'Neill Herbal Remedies

Uva Ursi (Arctostaphylos uva-ursi): Uva ursi is commonly used to treat urinary tract infections (UTIs). It has antiseptic properties that help cleanse the urinary tract. Uva ursi can be taken as a tea or in capsule form, but it should be used under the guidance of a healthcare professional due to potential side effects with prolonged use.

Cranberry (Vaccinium macrocarpon): Cranberry is well-known for its ability to prevent and treat UTIs by preventing bacteria from adhering to the urinary tract walls. Cranberry juice, extract, or capsules are common forms of consumption.

Vitex (Vitex agnus-castus): In addition to its benefits for PMS, vitex can be helpful for conditions like polycystic ovary syndrome (PCOS) by promoting hormonal balance. Usually, it is taken in the form of a capsule or tincture.

Ashwagandha (Withania somnifera): Ashwagandha is an adaptogen that helps the body manage stress and supports overall hormonal balance. It can be beneficial for women experiencing adrenal fatigue or stress-related hormonal imbalances. Ashwagandha is available as a powder, capsule, or tincture.

Barbara O'Neill Herbal Remedies

General Wellness and Hormonal Balance

Maintaining overall wellness and hormonal balance is essential for women's health. Here are some herbs that support these goals:

Maca (Lepidium meyenii): Maca is known for its ability to balance hormones, increase energy, and enhance libido. It can be particularly helpful for women experiencing symptoms of hormonal imbalances, such as irregular periods or menopausal symptoms. Maca powder can be added to smoothies or taken as a capsule.

Holy Basil (Ocimum sanctum): Holy basil, also known as tulsi, is an adaptogen that helps the body cope with stress and supports hormonal balance. It can be consumed as a pill, tincture, or tea.

Dandelion (Taraxacum officinale): Dandelion supports liver health, which is crucial for hormone regulation. It also acts as a gentle diuretic, helping to reduce water retention and bloating. Dandelion root tea or capsules are common forms of consumption.

Barbara O'Neill Herbal Remedies

CHAPTER NINE

MEN'S HEALTH

Men's health encompasses a range of issues from sexual health and vitality to cardiovascular wellness and prostate care. Herbal remedies offer natural, effective solutions to support men's health at various stages of life. This chapter explores various herbs that can help address common men's health concerns and provides practical guidance for their use.

Sexual Health and Vitality

Maintaining sexual health and vitality is important for overall well-being. Herbal remedies can help enhance libido, improve erectile function, and boost energy levels.

Ginseng (Panax ginseng): Ginseng is renowned for its ability to enhance energy, reduce fatigue, and improve sexual function. It can help with erectile dysfunction and boost libido. Ginseng is typically taken as a supplement or in tea form.

Maca (Lepidium meyenii): Maca is known for its ability to balance hormones and enhance libido. It can also improve stamina and energy levels. Maca powder can be added to smoothies or taken as a

Barbara O'Neill Herbal Remedies

capsule.

Tribulus (Tribulus terrestris): Tribulus is commonly used to enhance libido and improve sexual function. It is believed to increase testosterone levels and support overall sexual health. Tribulus is available as a supplement.

Horny Goat Weed (Epimedium spp.): Horny goat weed is traditionally used to improve erectile function and increase libido. It works by increasing blood flow to the sexual organs. As a supplement, it is OK.

Prostate Health

Men should take care of their prostates, especially as they get older. Herbal remedies can help prevent and manage conditions such as benign prostatic hyperplasia (BPH) and prostatitis.

Saw Palmetto (Serenoa repens): Saw palmetto is widely used to support prostate health and alleviate symptoms of BPH, such as frequent urination and difficulty urinating. It works by inhibiting the enzyme that converts testosterone into dihydrotestosterone (DHT), which can contribute to prostate enlargement. Saw palmetto is available as a supplement, tincture, or tea.

Pygeum (Pygeum africanum): Pygeum extract is derived from the bark of the African cherry tree and is used to treat urinary symptoms

Barbara O'Neill Herbal Remedies

associated with BPH. It has anti-inflammatory properties that help reduce prostate swelling. Pygeum can be taken as a capsule or tincture.

Nettle Root (Urtica dioica): Nettle root is beneficial for prostate health and can help reduce symptoms of BPH. When combined with saw palmetto, it functions nicely. Nettle root extract is available as a supplement or tincture.

Pumpkin Seed (Cucurbita pepo): Pumpkin seeds and their oil are rich in zinc and other nutrients that support prostate health. They help reduce inflammation and improve urinary function. Pumpkin seed oil can be taken as a supplement, or the seeds can be eaten as a snack.

Hormonal Balance and Vitality

Maintaining hormonal balance is essential for overall vitality and well-being. Herbal remedies can support energy levels, libido, and general hormonal health.

- **Ashwagandha (Withania somnifera)**: Ashwagandha is an adaptogen that helps the body manage stress and supports overall hormonal balance. It can enhance energy, stamina,

Barbara O'Neill Herbal Remedies

and libido. Ashwagandha is available as a powder, capsule, or tincture.

- **Tribulus (Tribulus terrestris)**: Tribulus is often used to boost testosterone levels and enhance libido. It supports overall hormonal balance and vitality. Tribulus can be taken as a supplement or tincture.

- **Maca (Lepidium meyenii)**: Maca is known for its ability to balance hormones and increase energy and libido. It can be particularly beneficial for men experiencing symptoms of low testosterone or hormonal imbalances. Maca powder can be added to smoothies or taken as a capsule.

- **Ginseng (Panax ginseng)**: Ginseng is an adaptogen that supports energy, stamina, and overall vitality. It is also known to improve sexual health and libido. Ginseng can be taken as a tea, supplement, or tincture.

Sexual Health

Herbal remedies can support sexual health, improving libido, performance, and overall satisfaction.

Horny Goat Weed (Epimedium spp.): Horny goat weed is traditionally used to enhance libido and improve erectile function. It

Barbara O'Neill Herbal Remedies

works by increasing blood flow and supporting healthy sexual function. Horny goat weed is available as a supplement or tincture.

Yohimbe (Pausinystalia yohimbe): Yohimbe bark extract is known for its ability to enhance libido and improve erectile function. It improves the vaginal area's blood flow. Yohimbe should be used with caution and under the guidance of a healthcare professional due to potential side effects.

Muira Puama (Ptychopetalum olacoides): Muira puama, also known as "potency wood," is used to enhance libido and improve sexual performance. It is available as a supplement or tincture.

Ginkgo Biloba (Ginkgo biloba): Ginkgo biloba improves blood flow and can enhance sexual function and libido. It also promotes general energy and cognitive function. Ginkgo can be taken as a supplement, tincture, or tea.

Stress Management and Mental Health

Managing stress and maintaining mental health are crucial aspects of overall well-being. Herbal remedies can help reduce stress, anxiety, and depression, promoting a sense of calm and balance.

Rhodiola (Rhodiola rosea): Rhodiola is an adaptogen that helps the body cope with stress and supports mental clarity and energy. It might lessen weariness and enhance general wellbeing. Rhodiola is

Barbara O'Neill Herbal Remedies

available as a supplement or tincture.

Holy Basil (Ocimum sanctum): Holy basil, also known as tulsi, is an adaptogen that helps manage stress and supports mental health. It has calming properties and can improve mood. Holy basil can be taken as a tea, tincture, or supplement.

St. John's Wort (Hypericum perforatum): St. John's wort is frequently used to treat anxiety and mild to moderate depression. It supports overall mental health and well-being. St. John's wort is available as a tea, tincture, or capsule.

Valerian (Valeriana officinalis): Valerian root is known for its calming effects and is used to treat anxiety and insomnia. It promotes relaxation and improves sleep quality. Valerian can be taken as a tea, tincture, or capsule.

Barbara O'Neill Herbal Remedies
CHAPTER TEN

Mental and Emotional Well-being

Mental and emotional well-being are fundamental to a healthy and fulfilling life. Stress, anxiety, depression, and other emotional challenges can significantly impact overall health. Herbal remedies offer natural and effective ways to support mental clarity, reduce stress, and promote emotional balance. This chapter explores various herbs that can enhance mental and emotional well-being and provides practical advice for their use.

Stress Management

Managing stress is crucial for maintaining mental and physical health. Herbal remedies can help the body cope with stress and reduce its negative impact.

Ashwagandha (Withania somnifera): Ashwagandha is an adaptogen that helps the body manage stress and supports overall well-being. It reduces cortisol levels and promotes a sense of calm. Ashwagandha is available as a powder, capsule, or tincture.

Rhodiola (Rhodiola rosea): Rhodiola is another powerful

Barbara O'Neill Herbal Remedies

adaptogen that helps the body adapt to stress. It improves mental clarity, reduces fatigue, and enhances overall resilience. Rhodiola can be taken as a supplement or tincture.

Holy Basil (Ocimum sanctum): Holy basil, also known as tulsi, has adaptogenic properties that help reduce stress and promote emotional balance. It can improve mood and mental clarity. Holy basil can be taken as a tea, tincture, or supplement.

Eleuthero (Eleutherococcus senticosus): Also known as Siberian ginseng, eleuthero helps the body handle stress and supports mental and physical endurance. It can be taken as a supplement or tincture.

Anxiety Relief

Herbs can offer a natural way to reduce anxiety and promote a sense of calm and relaxation.

Lavender (Lavandula angustifolia): Lavender is well-known for its calming and relaxing properties. It can help reduce anxiety and improve sleep quality. Lavender can be used as an essential oil, tea, or in bath products.

Passionflower (Passiflora incarnata): Passionflower is used to treat anxiety and insomnia. It promotes relaxation and can help calm the mind. Passionflower is available as a tea, tincture, or supplement.

Lemon Balm (Melissa officinalis): Lemon balm has calming effects

Barbara O'Neill Herbal Remedies

that can help reduce anxiety and improve mood. It is gentle and safe for regular use. Lemon balm can be taken as a tea, tincture, or supplement.

Valerian (Valeriana officinalis): Valerian root is effective for treating anxiety and promoting relaxation. It is also used to improve sleep quality. It can be consumed as a pill, tincture, or tea.

Mood Enhancement

Certain herbs can help improve mood and alleviate symptoms of depression, promoting a more positive emotional state.

St. John's Wort (Hypericum perforatum): A typical treatment for mild to moderate depression is St. John's wort. It supports overall mental health and well-being. St. John's wort is available as a tea, tincture, or capsule.

Saffron (Crocus sativus): Saffron has mood-enhancing properties and has been shown to be effective in treating mild depression. Saffron can be taken as a supplement or used in cooking.

Damiana (Turnera diffusa): Damiana is used to improve mood and reduce symptoms of mild depression and anxiety. It can also enhance libido and overall well-being. Damiana is available as a tea, tincture, or supplement.

Ginkgo Biloba (Ginkgo biloba): Ginkgo biloba improves

Barbara O'Neill Herbal Remedies

circulation to the brain and can help enhance mood and cognitive function. It supports overall mental clarity and well-being. Ginkgo can be taken as a supplement, tincture, or tea.

Cognitive Support

Maintaining cognitive function and mental clarity is essential for overall mental well-being. Herbs can support brain health and improve cognitive performance.

Ginkgo Biloba (Ginkgo biloba): Ginkgo biloba is one of the best-known herbs for supporting cognitive function. It improves blood flow to the brain, enhancing memory and mental clarity. Ginkgo can be taken as a supplement, tincture, or tea.

Bacopa (Bacopa monnieri): Bacopa is an herb used in Ayurvedic medicine to enhance cognitive function and improve memory. It also helps reduce anxiety and stress. Bacopa can be taken as a supplement or tincture.

Rosemary (Rosmarinus officinalis): Rosemary has been shown to improve memory and cognitive performance. It can be used in cooking, as an essential oil, or as a tea.

Gotu Kola (Centella asiatica): Gotu kola is another herb used in Ayurvedic medicine to support cognitive function and mental clarity. It helps improve memory and reduce anxiety. Gotu kola can be taken

Barbara O'Neill Herbal Remedies

as a tea, tincture, or supplement.

Sleep Support

Good quality sleep is crucial for mental and emotional well-being. Herbal remedies can help improve sleep quality and promote restful sleep.

Chamomile (Matricaria chamomilla): Chamomile is a well-known herb for promoting relaxation and improving sleep quality. Chamomile tea is a popular bedtime drink to help unwind and prepare for sleep.

Valerian (Valeriana officinalis): Valerian root is effective in promoting restful sleep and treating insomnia. It can be consumed as a pill, tincture, or tea.

Hops (Humulus lupulus): Hops are commonly used to improve sleep quality and reduce anxiety. They can be taken as a tea, tincture, or supplement.

California Poppy (Eschscholzia californica): California poppy has mild sedative properties and can help promote relaxation and restful sleep. It is available as a tea, tincture, or supplement.

CHAPTER ELEVEN

BODY PAIN MANAGEMENT

Pain is a common issue that can arise from various conditions, including injuries, chronic illnesses, and inflammation. Herbal remedies offer natural and effective ways to manage pain without the side effects often associated with pharmaceutical options. This chapter explores various herbs that can help alleviate different types of pain and provides practical advice for their use.

Anti-Inflammatory Herbs

Inflammation is a common cause of pain, particularly in conditions such as arthritis and injuries. Anti-inflammatory herbs can help reduce inflammation and relieve pain.

Turmeric (Curcuma longa): This spice has a potent anti-inflammatory substance called curcumin. It is effective in reducing pain and inflammation in conditions such as arthritis. Turmeric can be taken as a supplement, tea, or added to food.

Ginger (Zingiber officinale): Ginger has potent anti-inflammatory and analgesic properties. It can help reduce pain and inflammation in conditions like arthritis and muscle soreness. Ginger can be taken as a tea, supplement, or used in cooking.

Boswellia (Boswellia serrata): Also known as Indian frankincense,

Barbara O'Neill Herbal Remedies

boswellia is effective in reducing inflammation and pain, particularly in arthritis. Boswellia can be taken as a supplement or tincture.

Willow Bark (Salix alba): Willow bark contains salicin, which is a natural precursor to aspirin. It has anti-inflammatory and analgesic properties, making it effective for reducing pain and inflammation. Willow bark can be taken as a tea, tincture, or supplement.

Muscle and Joint Pain

Herbs can help alleviate muscle and joint pain caused by overuse, injuries, or chronic conditions such as arthritis.

Arnica (Arnica montana): Arnica is widely used for its anti-inflammatory and pain-relieving properties. It is particularly effective for muscle pain, bruises, and sprains. Arnica is usually applied topically as a cream or ointment.

Devil's Claw (Harpagophytum procumbens): Devil's claw is effective in reducing pain and inflammation, particularly in conditions like arthritis and lower back pain. It can be taken as a supplement or tincture.

Cayenne (Capsicum annuum): Cayenne pepper contains capsaicin, which can help reduce pain by depleting substance P, a chemical involved in transmitting pain signals. Cayenne can be used topically as a cream or ointment for joint and muscle pain.

Comfrey (Symphytum officinale): Comfrey is known for its ability

Barbara O'Neill Herbal Remedies

to promote healing and reduce pain. It is particularly effective for bruises, sprains, and muscle injuries. Comfrey is typically used topically as a cream or poultice.

Headache and Migraine Relief

Certain herbs can help alleviate headaches and migraines by reducing inflammation, improving circulation, and relaxing tension.

Feverfew(Tanacetum parthenium): Feverfew is commonly used to prevent and reduce the severity of migraines. It helps reduce inflammation and relax blood vessels in the brain. Feverfew can be taken as a tea, supplement, or tincture.

Peppermint (Mentha piperita): Peppermint has analgesic and cooling properties that can help relieve tension headaches. Peppermint oil can be applied topically to the temples and forehead, or peppermint tea can be consumed.

Butterbur (Petasites hybridus): Butterbur is effective in reducing the frequency and severity of migraines. It works by reducing inflammation and spasms in blood vessels. Butterbur can be taken as a supplement, but it should be used with caution and under the guidance of a healthcare professional due to potential liver toxicity.

Lavender(Lavandula angustifolia): Lavender has calming and analgesic properties that can help relieve headaches. Lavender

Barbara O'Neill Herbal Remedies

essential oil can be inhaled, applied topically, or used in a bath.

Chronic Pain Management

Chronic pain conditions, such as fibromyalgia and neuropathy, can significantly impact quality of life. Herbal treatments can provide comfort and enhance general health.

St. John's Wort (Hypericum perforatum): St. John's wort is effective in managing neuropathic pain and can also improve mood and emotional well-being. It can be consumed as a supplement, tincture, or tea.

Kava (Piper methysticum): Kava has muscle relaxant and analgesic properties that can help reduce chronic pain and improve relaxation. Kava can be taken as a tea, tincture, or supplement.

White Willow Bark (Salix alba): White willow bark is effective in managing chronic pain due to its anti-inflammatory and analgesic properties. It can be consumed as a supplement, tincture, or tea.

California Poppy (Eschscholzia California): California poppy is used to manage pain and promote relaxation. It has mild sedative properties and can be taken as a tea, tincture, or supplement.

Barbara O'Neill Herbal Remedies

Topical Pain Relief

Topical applications of herbs can provide direct pain relief to the affected area, offering a natural alternative to over-the-counter creams and ointments.

Menthol (Mentha spp.): Menthol provides a cooling sensation that can help relieve pain from muscle aches and joint pain. It is commonly used in topical pain relief products.

Capsaicin (Capsicum annuum): Capsaicin, derived from cayenne pepper, can be used topically to relieve pain by reducing substance P in the body. It is available in creams and ointments.

Eucalyptus (Eucalyptus globulus): Eucalyptus oil has anti-inflammatory and analgesic properties. It can be applied topically to reduce pain and inflammation in muscles and joints.

Comfrey (Symphytum officinale): Comfrey can be applied topically to reduce pain and promote healing of bruises, sprains, and muscle injuries. It is available in creams, ointments, and poultices.

CHAPTER TWELVE

CARDIOVASCULAR HEALTH

Cardiovascular health is crucial for maintaining overall well-being and preventing serious conditions such as heart disease, hypertension, and stroke. Herbs have been used traditionally to support heart health, improve circulation, and manage blood pressure and cholesterol levels. This chapter explores a variety of herbs that can contribute to cardiovascular health and offers practical advice on their use.

Supporting Heart Health

Keeping the heart healthy is crucial for overall cardiovascular health. Certain herbs can strengthen heart function and support overall cardiovascular health.

Hawthorn (Crataegus spp.): Hawthorn is renowned for its heart-strengthening properties. It improves blood flow to the heart, supports healthy blood pressure levels, and reduces symptoms of heart failure. Hawthorn can be taken as a tea, tincture, or supplement. Regular use can help enhance heart function and reduce angina symptoms.

Garlic (Allium sativum): Garlic is well-known for its cardiovascular benefits. It helps lower blood pressure, reduce cholesterol levels, and improve overall heart health. Garlic can be consumed fresh, in capsules, or as a tincture. Its active compounds, such as allicin, contribute to its heart-protective effects.

Olive Leaf (Olea europaea): Olive leaf extract supports cardiovascular health by improving blood circulation and reducing blood pressure. It has antioxidant and anti-inflammatory properties that contribute to heart health. Olive leaf extract can be taken as a supplement or in tea form.

Motherwort (Leonurus cardiaca): Motherwort is used to support heart health, particularly for symptoms such as palpitations and anxiety related to heart function. It has calming effects on the heart and can help manage blood pressure. Motherwort is available as a tea, tincture, or supplement.

Barbara O'Neill Herbal Remedies

Managing Blood Pressure

One of the main risk factors for cardiovascular disease is high blood pressure. Herbal remedies can help regulate and maintain healthy blood pressure levels.

Hawthorn (Crataegus spp.): In addition to its heart-strengthening properties, hawthorn is effective in managing high blood pressure. It helps dilate blood vessels and improve circulation. Hawthorn can be used as a tea, tincture, or supplement.

Garlic (Allium sativum): Garlic has been shown to have blood pressure-lowering effects. Its active ingredients facilitate improved blood flow and blood vessel relaxation. Garlic can be consumed raw, in capsules, or as a tincture.

Celery Seed (Apium graveolens): Celery seed is used to reduce high blood pressure and support kidney function. It acts as a diuretic and helps to lower blood pressure. Celery seed can be taken as a supplement or in tea form.

Linden Flower (Tilia spp.): Linden flower is known for its ability to help lower blood pressure and promote relaxation. It has mild diuretic and vasodilatory effects. You can drink linden flower tea or tincture.

Cholesterol Management

Maintaining healthy cholesterol levels is important for preventing

Barbara O'Neill Herbal Remedies

cardiovascular diseases. Herbal remedies can support healthy cholesterol levels and improve overall heart health.

Red Clover (Trifolium pratense): Red clover contains compounds that help reduce cholesterol levels and improve cardiovascular health. It also has antioxidant properties. You can consume red clover as a supplement, tincture, or tea.

Guggul (Commiphora wightii): Guggul is used in Ayurvedic medicine to manage cholesterol levels and support overall heart health. It aids in raising HDL (good) cholesterol and lowering LDL (bad) cholesterol. You can take guggul as a dietary supplement.

Psyllium (Plantago ovata): Psyllium is a source of soluble fiber that helps lower cholesterol levels and support heart health. It can be taken as a supplement or added to food.

Artichoke Leaf (Cynara scolymus): Artichoke leaf extract supports healthy cholesterol levels by promoting bile production and reducing cholesterol absorption. It can be taken as a supplement or in tea form.

Improving Circulation

Good circulation is vital for heart health and overall well-being. Certain herbs can help improve blood flow and support vascular health.

Barbara O'Neill Herbal Remedies

Ginkgo Biloba (Ginkgo biloba): Ginkgo biloba improves blood flow by dilating blood vessels and reducing blood viscosity. It supports cardiovascular health and enhances cognitive function. Ginkgo can be taken as a supplement, tincture, or tea.

Cayenne (Capsicum annuum): Cayenne pepper contains capsaicin, which helps improve circulation and reduce blood clotting. It supports overall cardiovascular health and can be taken as a supplement, tincture, or added to food.

Horse Chestnut (Aesculus hippocastanum): Horse chestnut supports healthy circulation and vein function, particularly in cases of chronic venous insufficiency. It helps reduce swelling and improve blood flow. Horse chestnut can be taken as a supplement or tincture.

Bilberry (Vaccinium myrtillus): Bilberry is used to support vascular health and improve circulation. It contains antioxidants that help strengthen blood vessels and improve capillary function. Bilberry can be taken as a supplement or in tea form.

General Cardiovascular Support

In addition to targeting specific cardiovascular issues, certain herbs provide general support for heart health and overall cardiovascular function.

Turmeric (Curcuma longa): Turmeric has anti-inflammatory and

Barbara O'Neill Herbal Remedies

antioxidant properties that support cardiovascular health. It helps reduce inflammation and oxidative stress, contributing to heart health. Turmeric can be taken as a supplement, tea, or added to food.

Coenzyme Q10 (CoQ10): While not an herb, CoQ10 is a naturally occurring antioxidant that supports heart health by improving energy production in heart cells and reducing oxidative stress. One can purchase CoQ10 as a nutritional supplement.

Green Tea (Camellia sinensis): Green tea contains antioxidants called catechins that support cardiovascular health by improving blood vessel function and reducing cholesterol levels. Green tea can be consumed as a beverage or taken as a supplement.

In conclusion, herbal remedies offer a range of benefits for cardiovascular health, from supporting heart function and managing blood pressure to improving circulation and cholesterol levels. By incorporating these herbs into your routine, you can promote overall cardiovascular well-being and reduce the risk of heart-related conditions. Before beginning any new herbal regimen, always get medical advice, especially if you have pre-existing health concerns or are currently taking medicine.

Barbara O'Neill Herbal Remedies

CHAPTER THIRTEEN

DIABETES AND BLOOD SUGAR CONTROL

Diabetes and blood sugar control are critical aspects of maintaining overall health, particularly for individuals with diabetes or those at risk of developing it. Managing blood sugar levels effectively can prevent complications and improve quality of life. Herbal remedies can play a supportive role in blood sugar regulation, complementing conventional treatments. This chapter explores various herbs that help manage blood sugar levels and support metabolic health.

Herbs for Blood Sugar Regulation

Several herbs have been shown to help regulate blood sugar levels and improve insulin sensitivity, making them valuable tools for managing diabetes.

Cinnamon (Cinnamomum spp.): Cinnamon is well-known for its ability to improve insulin sensitivity and lower blood sugar levels. It helps enhance glucose uptake by cells and can be a beneficial addition to a diabetes management plan. Cinnamon can be added to food, taken as a supplement, or consumed in tea form.

Barbara O'Neill Herbal Remedies

Fenugreek (Trigonella foenum-graecum): Fenugreek seeds are rich in soluble fiber and have been shown to help lower blood sugar levels and improve insulin sensitivity. Fenugreek can be taken as a supplement, in powder form, or used in cooking.

Bitter Melon (Momordica charantia): Bitter melon contains compounds that mimic insulin and help lower blood sugar levels. It can also improve glucose metabolism. Bitter melon can be consumed as a juice, supplement, or added to food.

Gymnema (Gymnema sylvestre): Gymnema is traditionally used in Ayurvedic medicine to manage diabetes. It helps reduce sugar absorption in the intestines and can improve insulin function. Gymnema is available as a supplement or tincture.

Herbs for Enhancing Insulin Sensitivity

Improving insulin sensitivity is crucial for managing blood sugar levels and preventing insulin resistance.

Berberine (Berberis spp.): Berberine is a potent compound found in several herbs, including goldenseal and barberry. It helps improve insulin sensitivity, reduce blood sugar levels, and support overall metabolic health. Berberine is available as a supplement and can be particularly effective in managing type 2 diabetes.

Alpha-Lipoic Acid (ALA): Though not an herb, alpha-lipoic acid is

Barbara O'Neill Herbal Remedies

a powerful antioxidant that supports insulin sensitivity and helps manage blood sugar levels. It can be taken as a supplement to complement herbal treatments.

Ginseng (Panax ginseng): Panax ginseng has been shown to improve insulin sensitivity and help regulate blood sugar levels. It also provides energy and reduces fatigue. Ginseng can be taken as a supplement, tea, or tincture.

Astragalus (Astragalus membranaceus): Astragalus supports overall immune function and has been shown to help manage blood sugar levels. It improves insulin sensitivity and can be taken as a supplement or tincture.

Herbs for Reducing Complications

Managing diabetes involves preventing and treating complications such as neuropathy, cardiovascular issues, and inflammation.

Turmeric (Curcuma longa): Turmeric contains curcumin, which has anti-inflammatory and antioxidant properties. It helps reduce inflammation and oxidative stress associated with diabetes complications. Turmeric can be taken as a supplement, tea, or added to food.

Ginger (Zingiber officinale): Ginger has anti-inflammatory and antioxidant effects that can help manage diabetes-related

Barbara O'Neill Herbal Remedies

complications. It supports overall metabolic health and can be consumed as a tea, supplement, or used in cooking.

Nopal Cactus (Opuntia ficus-indica): Nopal cactus, also known as prickly pear, helps lower blood sugar levels and supports insulin sensitivity. It has also been shown to improve lipid profiles and reduce inflammation. Nopal can be consumed as a supplement, juice, or in its fresh form.

Holy Basil (Ocimum sanctum): Holy basil, or tulsi, helps reduce stress and inflammation, which can benefit individuals with diabetes. It also supports blood sugar regulation. Holy basil can be taken as a tea, supplement, or tincture.

General Blood Sugar Support

In addition to targeting specific aspects of diabetes management, some herbs provide general support for blood sugar control and metabolic health.

Dandelion (Taraxacum officinale): Dandelion supports liver health and has diuretic properties that can help manage blood sugar levels. It also promotes digestion and overall metabolic function. Dandelion can be consumed as a tea, supplement, or in its fresh form.

Mulberry (Morus alba): Mulberry leaves have been traditionally used to manage blood sugar levels. They contain compounds that

Barbara O'Neill Herbal Remedies

inhibit carbohydrate absorption and improve insulin sensitivity. Mulberry can be taken as a supplement or tea.

Coriander (Coriandrum sativum): Coriander has been shown to support blood sugar regulation and improve metabolic health. It can be consumed as a supplement or utilized in cookery.

Bilberry (Vaccinium myrtillus): Bilberry supports vascular health and improves blood glucose control. It contains antioxidants that help reduce oxidative stress and improve insulin function. Bilberry can be taken as a supplement or in tea form.

Considerations and Cautions

While herbal remedies can be beneficial, it's important to use them as a complementary approach alongside conventional treatments. Always consult with a healthcare professional before starting any new herbal regimen, especially if you have existing health conditions, are taking other medications, or are managing diabetes. Some herbs may interact with medications or have side effects, so professional guidance ensures safe and effective use.

In conclusion, herbal remedies offer valuable support for managing diabetes and blood sugar levels. By incorporating these herbs into your routine, you can improve insulin sensitivity, regulate blood sugar levels, and support overall metabolic health.

CHAPTER 14

DETOXIFICATION AND CLEANSING

Detoxification and cleansing are processes aimed at removing toxins from the body and supporting overall health. While the body naturally detoxifies through the liver, kidneys, and digestive system, herbal remedies can enhance these processes and promote well-being. This chapter explores various herbs that support detoxification and cleansing, helping to rejuvenate the body and maintain optimal health.

Supporting Liver Health.

The liver is the primary organ responsible for detoxification, processing toxins, and metabolizing nutrients. Herbs that support liver function can enhance the body's natural detoxification processes.

Milk Thistle (Silybum marianum): Milk thistle is renowned for its liver-protective properties. Its active compound, silymarin, supports liver cell regeneration, protects against toxins, and improves liver function. Milk thistle can be taken as a supplement, tincture, or tea.

Dandelion Root (Taraxacum officinale): Dandelion root supports liver health by stimulating bile production and promoting

Barbara O'Neill Herbal Remedies

detoxification. It also acts as a gentle diuretic, aiding in the elimination of toxins through the urinary system. Dandelion root can be consumed as a tea, supplement, or tincture.

Artichoke (Cynara scolymus): Artichoke has been shown to support liver function and promote bile production, aiding in digestion and detoxification. Artichoke extract can be taken as a supplement or consumed as a tea.

Turmeric (Curcuma longa): Turmeric, particularly its active compound curcumin, has anti-inflammatory and antioxidant effects that support liver health and detoxification. Turmeric can be added to meals, taken as a supplement, or eaten as a tea.

Enhancing Kidney Function

In order to filter blood and eliminate waste from the body, the kidneys are essential. Supporting kidney function can enhance detoxification and overall health.

Nettle (Urtica dioica): Nettle is a natural diuretic that helps support kidney function and promotes the elimination of excess fluids and toxins. It also has anti-inflammatory properties that support overall kidney health. Nettle can be consumed as a tincture, tea, or supplement.

Cranberry (Vaccinium macrocarpon): Cranberry is well-known

Barbara O'Neill Herbal Remedies

for its role in urinary tract health and supports kidney function by promoting the elimination of waste products. Cranberry juice or supplements can be used to support kidney health.

Horsetail (Equisetum arvense): Horsetail has diuretic properties that support kidney function and enhance the elimination of toxins through urine. It can be consumed as a supplement or tea.

Parsley (Petroselinum crispum): Parsley is a mild diuretic that supports kidney function and promotes detoxification. It can be used fresh in cooking, as a tea, or taken as a supplement.

Supporting Digestive Health

A healthy stomach is essential for a good detoxification process. Herbs that support digestion can enhance the body's ability to eliminate waste and toxins.

Ginger (Zingiber officinale): Ginger supports digestion by stimulating digestive enzymes and improving gut motility. It also has anti-inflammatory and antioxidant properties that support overall digestive health. Ginger can be consumed as a tea, supplement, or used in cooking.

Peppermint (Mentha piperita): Peppermint aids digestion by relaxing the muscles of the gastrointestinal tract and reducing symptoms of bloating and gas. Peppermint tea or oil can be used to

Barbara O'Neill Herbal Remedies

support digestive health.

Fennel (Foeniculum vulgare): Fennel supports digestion and reduces bloating and gas. Its carminative properties help ease digestive discomfort and promote healthy bowel function. Fennel can be consumed as a tea, in cooking, or taken as a supplement.

Aloe Vera (Aloe barbadensis): Aloe vera supports digestive health by promoting healthy bowel movements and reducing inflammation in the digestive tract. Aloe vera juice or supplements can be used to support digestive health.

Promoting Overall Detoxification

Several herbs support overall detoxification by enhancing the body's ability to eliminate toxins and improving general health.

Chlorella (Chlorella vulgaris): Chlorella is a green algae that helps detoxify the body by binding to heavy metals and other toxins and promoting their elimination. You can consume chlorella as a supplement.

Spirulina (Arthrospira platensis): Spirulina is another algae with detoxifying properties. It supports liver function, boosts energy, and helps eliminate toxins from the body. Spirulina can be taken as a supplement or powder.

Red Clover (Trifolium pratense): Red clover is known for its

Barbara O'Neill Herbal Remedies

detoxifying properties and supports lymphatic system function. It can help cleanse the blood and promote overall health. Red clover can be taken as a tea, supplement, or tincture.

Burdock Root (Arctium lappa): Burdock root supports liver and kidney function, promotes healthy digestion, and aids in detoxification. It can be consumed as a tea, supplement, or tincture.

General Considerations and Cautions

While herbal remedies can support detoxification and cleansing, it is important to use them responsibly and as part of a balanced approach to health. Before beginning any new herbal regimen, always get medical advice, especially if you have pre-existing health concerns or are currently taking medicine.

Some herbs may interact with medications or have side effects, so professional guidance ensures safe and effective use.

In conclusion, herbal remedies offer valuable support for detoxification and cleansing, enhancing the body's natural processes and promoting overall health. By incorporating these herbs into your routine, you can support liver and kidney function, improve digestive health, and promote general detoxification.

Barbara O'Neill Herbal Remedies

CHAPTER FIFTEEN

BONE AND JOINT HEALTH

Maintaining bone and joint health is essential for mobility, strength, and overall quality of life. As we age, bone density can decrease, and joints can become susceptible to wear and tear, leading to conditions such as osteoporosis and arthritis. Herbal remedies can support bone density, reduce inflammation, and alleviate joint pain, contributing to overall skeletal health. This chapter explores various herbs known for their beneficial effects on bone and joint health.

Supporting Bone Health

Herbs that support bone health can help maintain bone density and prevent conditions such as osteoporosis.

Horsetail (Equisetum arvense): Horsetail is rich in silica, a mineral that supports bone health by promoting collagen formation and calcium absorption. Silica strengthens bones and connective tissues, making horsetail a valuable herb for maintaining bone density. Horsetail can be taken as a tea, tincture, or supplement.

Nettle (Urtica dioica): Nettle is high in minerals such as calcium, magnesium, and iron, which are essential for bone health. It supports overall bone strength and helps prevent bone loss. Nettle can be

Barbara O'Neill Herbal Remedies

consumed as a tea, supplement, or in its fresh form.

Red Clover (Trifolium pratense): Red clover contains phytoestrogens that can help maintain bone density, especially in postmenopausal women. It supports overall skeletal health and can be taken as a tea, supplement, or tincture.

Alfalfa (Medicago sativa): Alfalfa is rich in vitamins and minerals, including calcium and magnesium, which are crucial for bone health. It can be taken as a supplement or consumed as a tea.

Reducing Inflammation and Supporting Joint Health

Herbs that reduce inflammation and support joint health can help alleviate pain and improve mobility in conditions such as arthritis.

Turmeric (Curcuma longa): Turmeric, particularly its active compound curcumin, has potent anti-inflammatory properties that can help reduce joint pain and inflammation. Turmeric can be taken as a supplement, added to food, or consumed as a tea.

Ginger (Zingiber officinale): Ginger has anti-inflammatory and analgesic properties that help reduce joint pain and inflammation. It can be consumed as a tea, supplement, or used in cooking.

Boswellia (Boswellia serrata): Boswellia, also known as Indian frankincense, contains boswellic acids that have powerful anti-inflammatory effects. It can help reduce pain and improve joint

Barbara O'Neill Herbal Remedies

function in conditions like osteoarthritis. Boswellia can be taken as a supplement or tincture.

Devil's Claw (Harpagophytum procumbens): Devil's Claw is known for its anti-inflammatory and analgesic properties, making it effective in reducing joint pain and improving mobility. It can be consumed as a tincture or supplement.

Willow Bark (Salix alba): Willow bark contains salicin, a compound similar to aspirin, and has been used for centuries to reduce pain and inflammation. It can be consumed as a supplement or tea.

Promoting Cartilage Health

Supporting cartilage health is crucial for maintaining joint function and preventing degenerative joint conditions.

Cat's Claw (Uncaria tomentosa): Cat's Claw has anti-inflammatory properties and supports the immune system. It can help reduce joint inflammation and support cartilage health. It can be consumed as a tincture or supplement.

Ashwagandha (Withania somnifera): Ashwagandha has adaptogenic and anti-inflammatory properties that support joint health and reduce pain. It can also help improve overall physical function. Ashwagandha can be taken as a supplement or tincture.

Barbara O'Neill Herbal Remedies

Licorice Root (Glycyrrhiza glabra): Licorice root has anti-inflammatory properties that can help reduce joint pain and support cartilage health. It can be taken as a tea, supplement, or tincture.

Stinging Nettle (Urtica dioica): Nettle has anti-inflammatory properties and is rich in minerals essential for joint and cartilage health. It can be consumed as a tea, supplement, or in its fresh form.

General Considerations and Cautions

While herbal remedies can support bone and joint health, they should be used as part of a comprehensive approach to health, including a balanced diet, regular exercise, and proper medical care. Before beginning any new herbal regimen, always get medical advice, especially if you have pre-existing health concerns or are currently taking medicine. Some herbs may interact with medications or have side effects, so professional guidance ensures safe and effective use.

In conclusion, herbal remedies offer valuable support for maintaining bone and joint health. By incorporating these herbs into your routine, you can improve bone density, reduce inflammation, alleviate joint pain, and support overall skeletal health.

CHAPTER SIXTEEN

CREATING A HERBAL MEDICINE CABINET

A well-stocked herbal medicine cabinet can provide natural remedies for a variety of common ailments and support overall health. By keeping essential herbs and herbal preparations on hand, you can address minor health issues quickly and effectively. This chapter guides you through selecting key herbs and herbal preparations to create a versatile and effective herbal medicine cabinet.

Essential Herbs and Their Uses

Here are some foundational herbs that should be included in any herbal medicine cabinet, along with their primary uses.

Chamomile (Matricaria chamomilla): Known for its calming and anti-inflammatory properties, chamomile is useful for promoting relaxation, soothing digestive issues, and reducing skin irritation. It can be used as a tea, tincture, or topical application.

Peppermint (Mentha piperita): Peppermint is excellent for digestive health, relieving headaches, and easing muscle tension. It can be used as a tea, tincture, essential oil, or in a topical balm.

Echinacea (Echinacea purpurea): Echinacea supports the immune

Barbara O'Neill Herbal Remedies

system and can help shorten the duration of colds and flu. It can be consumed as a pill, tincture, or tea.

Ginger (Zingiber officinale): Ginger is effective for nausea, digestive issues, and inflammation. It can be used fresh, as a tea, tincture, or in capsule form.

Lavender (Lavandula angustifolia): Lavender is known for its calming effects and is useful for stress relief, sleep support, and skin irritations. It can be used as an essential oil, in teas, or as a topical application.

Turmeric (Curcuma longa): Turmeric has powerful anti-inflammatory properties and can support joint health and overall inflammation reduction. It can be taken as a powder, in capsules, or as a tea.

Garlic (Allium sativum): Garlic has antimicrobial and immune-boosting properties and is useful for infections and cardiovascular health. It can be taken fresh, in capsules, or as an oil.

Calendula (Calendula officinalis): Calendula is excellent for skin healing, minor cuts, and inflammations. It can be used as an infused oil, in salves, or as a tea.

Thyme (Thymus vulgaris): Thyme has strong antimicrobial properties and is useful for respiratory issues and infections. It can be used as a tea, tincture, or essential oil.

Barbara O'Neill Herbal Remedies

St. John's Wort (Hypericum perforatum): St. John's Wort is beneficial for mood support and minor skin irritations. It can be taken as a tea, tincture, or in oil form.

Herbal Preparations and Their Uses

Understanding different forms of herbal preparations can help you use herbs effectively.

Teas (Infusions and Decoctions): Teas are a simple way to extract the beneficial compounds from herbs. Infusions are made by steeping leaves and flowers in hot water, while decoctions involve simmering harder parts like roots and bark.

Tinctures: Herbs are soaked in glycerin or alcohol to create concentrated liquid extracts known as tinctures. They are potent and convenient, requiring only a few drops to be effective.

Capsules and Tablets: Herbal capsules and tablets provide a convenient way to consume herbs, especially those with strong flavors or when precise dosing is needed.

Essential Oils: Essential oils are highly concentrated extracts used primarily for aromatherapy and topical applications. They should be diluted before use.

Salves and Balms: These are ointments made by infusing herbs in

Barbara O'Neill Herbal Remedies

oils and combining them with beeswax or other thickening agents. They are excellent for skin conditions and localized pain relief.

Syrups: Herbal syrups are made by combining herbal decoctions or infusions with honey or sugar. They are particularly useful for soothing coughs and sore throats.

Poultices and Compresses: These are used for direct application to the skin, where herbs are mashed or infused and applied to the affected area to reduce inflammation or draw out infections.

Setting Up Your Herbal Medicine Cabinet

Organizing your herbal medicine cabinet efficiently can make it easier to find and use the remedies you need.

Storage: Keep herbs and herbal preparations in a cool, dark place to maintain their potency. Use airtight containers to prevent moisture and light from degrading the herbs.

Labeling: Clearly label all containers with the herb name, preparation type, and date of preparation. This helps ensure you use the herbs before they lose their efficacy.

Safety: Store herbs and preparations out of reach of children and pets. Ensure you have a clear understanding of each herb's uses and potential side effects.

Barbara O'Neill Herbal Remedies

Basic Tools: Equip your herbal medicine cabinet with basic tools such as measuring spoons, droppers, tea infusers, and mortar and pestle for preparing and using your herbal remedies.

Herbal First Aid Kit

In addition to your herbal medicine cabinet, consider creating a smaller, portable herbal first aid kit for travel and emergencies.

Arnica Gel/Cream: For bruises and muscle aches.

Lavender Essential Oil: For stress relief, sleep support, and minor burns.

Calendula Salve: For cuts, scrapes, and skin irritations.

Activated Charcoal: For food poisoning and detoxification.

Echinacea Tincture: For immune support.

Peppermint Essential Oil: For headaches and digestive issues.

Ginger Capsules: For nausea and digestive support.

General Considerations and Cautions

While herbal remedies can be effective for many conditions, they should be used responsibly. Before beginning any new herbal regimen, always get medical advice, especially if you have pre-

Barbara O'Neill Herbal Remedies

existing health concerns or are currently taking medicine. Be aware of potential allergies and side effects, and use herbs according to recommended guidelines.

In conclusion, creating a well-stocked herbal medicine cabinet equips you with natural remedies for a variety of common ailments and supports overall health. By carefully selecting and organizing essential herbs and preparations, you can effectively manage minor health issues and promote well-being in a natural and holistic way.

CHAPTER SEVENTEEN

GROWING AND HARVESTING YOUR OWN HERBS

Cultivating your own herbs provides a fresh, convenient, and cost-effective way to have a steady supply of medicinal plants. Homegrown herbs ensure you have access to high-quality, chemical-free remedies and add a rewarding aspect to your herbal practice. This chapter guides you through the basics of growing, caring for, and harvesting your own herbs.

Choosing the Right Herbs

Start with herbs that are easy to grow and commonly used in herbal medicine.

Basil (Ocimum basilicum): Useful for its anti-inflammatory and digestive properties.

Chamomile (Matricaria chamomilla): Known for its calming effects and skin-healing properties.

Lavender (Lavandula angustifolia): Offers stress relief and sleep support.

Peppermint (Mentha piperita): Great for digestive issues and headaches.

Barbara O'Neill Herbal Remedies

Thyme (Thymus vulgaris): Has antimicrobial properties useful for respiratory issues.

Sage (Salvia officinalis): Beneficial for sore throats and digestive health.

Calendula (Calendula officinalis): Excellent for skin conditions and wound healing.

Echinacea (Echinacea purpurea): Supports the immune system.

Setting Up Your Herb Garden

Decide whether to grow your herbs indoors, outdoors, or both. Consider your available space, climate, and the specific needs of each herb.

Indoors: Ideal for herbs that require more controlled conditions. Use pots with good drainage, and place them in a sunny spot, such as a windowsill or under grow lights.

Outdoors: Suitable for herbs that thrive in natural conditions. Choose a sunny location with well-drained soil. Raised beds or garden plots work well.

Soil Preparation

Use well-draining, organic matter-rich soil for optimal soil quality. The quality of your soil can be raised by adding aged manure or

Barbara O'Neill Herbal Remedies

compost.

pH Level: Most herbs prefer a slightly acidic to neutral pH (6.0-7.0). Do a soil test and make any necessary amendments.

Planting Herbs

Seeds vs. Seedlings: Some herbs grow well from seeds, while others are better started from seedlings. Follow the specific planting instructions for each herb.

Spacing: Ensure adequate spacing between plants to allow for growth and airflow, which helps prevent disease.

Watering: Herbs generally prefer well-drained soil. Water them often, but don't give them too much, as this can cause root rot.

Caring for Your Herbs

Watering: Herbs typically need about an inch of water per week. Adjust based on rainfall and temperature.

Fertilizing: Use a balanced, organic fertilizer. Over-fertilizing can lead to excessive leaf growth with reduced medicinal properties.

Pruning: To promote bushy growth and keep herbs from growing lanky, regularly prune plants. Pruning also helps maintain the plant's shape and promotes more vigorous growth.

Barbara O'Neill Herbal Remedies

Pest and Disease Management

Natural Solutions: Apply natural pest management techniques including ladybug introduction, neem oil, and insecticidal soap.

Companion Planting: Plant herbs that repel pests near more vulnerable plants. For example, basil and marigolds can deter aphids and other common pests.

Monitoring: Keep an eye out for any indications of illness or pests on your plants. Maintaining healthy plants requires early detection and treatment.

Harvesting Herbs

Timing: Harvest herbs in the morning after the dew has dried but before the sun is too hot. This helps preserve the essential oils.

Frequency: Regular harvesting encourages more growth. For most herbs, it's best to harvest before the plants flower, as this is when they contain the highest concentration of medicinal compounds.

Method: Chop the herbs with pruning shears or sharp scissors. Don't pull or rip the plant since this could harm it.

Drying and Storing Herbs

Barbara O'Neill Herbal Remedies

Drying: Hang herbs in small bundles in a warm, dry, and dark place with good ventilation. As an alternative, use a low-temperature dehydrator.

Storage: Keep dried herbs in a cold, dark area in airtight containers.

Shelf Life: Most dried herbs retain their potency for about a year. Check for signs of mold or loss of color and aroma before use.

Using Fresh Herbs

Fresh herbs can be used immediately for teas, tinctures, and culinary purposes. The potency of fresh herbs is often higher than that of dried herbs, making them particularly effective in remedies.

General Considerations and Cautions

Identification: Ensure proper identification of herbs before consumption. Some plants may look similar but have different properties or toxicity levels.

Sustainability: Practice sustainable harvesting by not taking more than one-third of the plant at a time. As a result, the plant can keep developing and yielding.

Barbara O'Neill Herbal Remedies

CHAPTER EIGHTEEN

COOKING WITH HERBS

Incorporating herbs into your cooking not only enhances the flavor of your meals but also provides numerous health benefits. Culinary herbs are rich in vitamins, minerals, and antioxidants, and they offer a natural way to support digestion, boost the immune system, and promote overall well-being. This chapter explores various ways to use herbs in your cooking, from fresh salads to hearty soups and beyond.

Choosing the Right Herbs

Understanding the flavor profiles and health benefits of different herbs can help you select the right ones for your dishes.

Basil (Ocimum basilicum): Sweet and slightly peppery, basil is great in salads, pastas, and pesto. It has anti-inflammatory and antioxidant properties.

Rosemary (Rosmarinus officinalis): is aromatic and woodsy; it goes well with roasted vegetables and meats. It supports digestion and improves circulation.

Thyme (Thymus vulgaris): Earthy and slightly minty, thyme is versatile in soups, stews, and marinades. It has antimicrobial

Barbara O'Neill Herbal Remedies

properties and supports respiratory health.

Cilantro (Coriandrum sativum): Fresh and citrusy, cilantro is perfect for salsas, curries, and salads. It aids in detoxification and supports digestion.

Parsley (Petroselinum crispum): Mild and slightly peppery, parsley can be used in virtually any dish for a burst of freshness. It is rich in vitamins A, C, and K.

Mint (Mentha spp.): Refreshing and cool, mint is great in beverages, desserts, and salads. It aids digestion and has a calming effect.

Sage (Salvia officinalis): Earthy and slightly peppery, sage is ideal for stuffing, sauces, and roasted dishes. It supports digestive health and has anti-inflammatory properties.

Oregano (Origanum vulgare): Robust and slightly bitter, oregano is a staple in Mediterranean cuisine. It has antimicrobial properties and supports immune health.

Using Fresh Herbs

Fresh herbs add vibrant flavor and nutrients to dishes. Here are some pointers for making efficient use of them:

Preparation: Wash herbs thoroughly and pat them dry before use. Chop them finely or tear the leaves to release their essential oils.

Barbara O'Neill Herbal Remedies

Timing: Add delicate herbs like basil, cilantro, and parsley towards the end of cooking to preserve their flavor and nutrients. You can add hardier herbs, such thyme and rosemary, early in the cooking process.

Storage: Store fresh herbs in the refrigerator, wrapped in a damp paper towel and placed in a plastic bag, or in a glass of water like a bouquet.

Using Dried Herbs

Dried herbs are convenient and have a longer shelf life than fresh herbs. They are typically more concentrated, so adjust the quantities accordingly.

Conversion: As a general rule, use one-third the amount of dried herbs compared to fresh. For example, if a recipe calls for 3 teaspoons of fresh basil, use 1 teaspoon of dried basil.

Rehydration: To release their flavors, crush dried herbs between your fingers before adding them to your dishes. For soups and stews, you can add dried herbs directly; for other dishes, consider rehydrating them in a bit of hot water before use.

Storage: Keep dried herbs in a cold, dark area in airtight containers. They typically retain their potency for about a year.

Barbara O'Neill Herbal Remedies

Herbal Cooking Techniques

Integrate herbs into your cooking using various techniques:

Infused Oils and Vinegars: Create herb-infused oils and vinegars by steeping fresh or dried herbs in olive oil or vinegar. Use these infusions to dress salads, marinate meats, or drizzle over cooked vegetables.

Herb Butter: Make herb butter by blending softened butter with finely chopped fresh herbs. Use it to enhance the flavor of bread, vegetables, and grilled meats.

Pesto and Chimichurri: Blend fresh herbs like basil, cilantro, or parsley with garlic, nuts, olive oil, and cheese (for pesto) or vinegar (for chimichurri) to create flavorful sauces.

Herbal Salts: Mix dried herbs with coarse sea salt to create herbal salts. Use them to season meats, vegetables, and roasted dishes.

Herbal Teas: Prepare herbal teas by steeping fresh or dried herbs in hot water. Enjoy them as a beverage or use them as a flavorful base for soups and stews.

Recipes for Health-Boosting Meals

Here are some simple and delicious ways to incorporate herbs into your meals:

Herb Salad: Combine mixed greens with fresh herbs like basil,

Barbara O'Neill Herbal Remedies

parsley, and mint. Dress with herb-infused olive oil and lemon juice.

Herbed Roast Chicken: Rub a whole chicken with a mixture of chopped rosemary, thyme, garlic, and olive oil. Roast until golden and cooked through.

Minted Pea Soup: Sauté onions and garlic, add peas and vegetable broth, and simmer until tender. Blend with fresh mint and a splash of cream.

Pesto Pasta: Toss cooked pasta with fresh basil pesto and top with grated Parmesan cheese.

Roasted Potatoes with Rosemary: Combine potatoes, salt, pepper, and olive oil. Roast until crispy and golden.

Cilantro-Lime Rice: Cook rice with lime zest, and stir in chopped cilantro and lime juice before serving.

Barbara O'Neill Herbal Remedies

Infusing Oils and Vinegars

Infusing oils and vinegars with herbs is a simple yet powerful way to enhance the flavor and therapeutic properties of your culinary creations. These infusions not only add unique flavors to your dishes but also bring the health benefits of herbs into your kitchen.

Infusing Oils:

Method: To make herb-infused oils, fill a clean, dry glass jar with your chosen herbs (such as rosemary, thyme, or basil) and cover them with a high-quality oil like olive or grapeseed oil. Seal the jar and store it in a warm, dark place for 2-4 weeks. Shake the jar daily to help the herbs release their essential oils.

Straining and Storing: After the infusion period, strain out the herbs using a fine mesh strainer or cheesecloth. Transfer the infused oil to a clean, airtight bottle and store it in a cool, dark place. Infused oils can be used for cooking, salad dressings, or as a flavorful addition to various dishes.

Infusing Vinegars:

Method: To make herb-infused vinegars, place herbs (such as tarragon, dill, or cilantro) in a clean glass jar and cover them with your chosen vinegar (like apple cider or white wine vinegar). For two to four weeks, keep the jar sealed and placed in a cool, dark

Barbara O'Neill Herbal Remedies

spot. Shake the jar occasionally to mix the flavors.

Straining and Storing: After the infusion period, strain out the herbs using a fine mesh strainer or cheesecloth. Pour the infused vinegar into a clean, airtight bottle and store it in a cool, dark place. Infused vinegars can be used in salad dressings, marinades, or as a tangy flavor boost to dishes.

Tips:

Use dried herbs for infusions to reduce the risk of spoilage.

Always ensure that your jars and bottles are completely dry before use to prevent mold growth.

Experiment with different herb and oil or vinegar combinations to find your preferred flavors and benefits.

Infused oils and vinegars are versatile and easy to make, allowing you to enjoy the added benefits of herbs in your everyday cooking and personal wellness routines.

General Considerations and Cautions

While cooking with herbs is generally safe, be aware of any potential allergies or sensitivities. Start with small amounts if you're unfamiliar with a particular herb. Pregnant or breastfeeding women and individuals with specific health conditions should consult a healthcare professional before making significant dietary changes.

Barbara O'Neill Herbal Remedies

Conclusion

Herbal remedies offer a holistic and natural approach to health and wellness, harnessing the power of plants to support and enhance the body's innate healing abilities. Throughout this book, we have explored various aspects of herbal medicine, from understanding the basics to growing, harvesting, and using herbs in daily life. As we conclude, let's reflect on the key takeaways and the journey ahead.

Embracing a Holistic Approach

Herbal medicine is not just about treating symptoms; it is about supporting the whole person—body, mind, and spirit. Embracing a holistic approach means recognizing the interconnectedness of our health and well-being. By integrating herbal remedies with other healthy lifestyle practices, such as proper nutrition, regular exercise, and stress management, we can achieve a more balanced and harmonious state of health.

Empowerment Through Knowledge

One of the greatest benefits of herbal medicine is the empowerment it provides. By understanding the properties and uses of various herbs, you gain the knowledge to take control of your health naturally. This book has equipped you with the tools to identify, grow, harvest, and use herbs safely and effectively. As you continue

Barbara O'Neill Herbal Remedies

your herbal journey, keep learning, experimenting, and expanding your herbal repertoire.

Sustainability and Respect for Nature

Herbal medicine fosters a deep connection with nature. Growing your own herbs, harvesting them responsibly, and using them mindfully cultivates a sense of respect for the environment. Sustainable practices ensure that these valuable resources are available for future generations. Remember to honor the wisdom of traditional herbal knowledge while adapting it to modern needs in an ethical and environmentally conscious manner.

Personalization and Adaptability

Each person's health demands are distinct, just like them. Herbal remedies offer the flexibility to personalize your approach to health care. Listen to your body, observe how it responds to different herbs, and adapt your herbal practices accordingly. It's acceptable if something that works for one individual doesn't work for another. The key is to find what resonates with you and supports your individual health journey.

Seeking Professional Guidance

Barbara O'Neill Herbal Remedies

While herbal medicine is accessible and empowering, it is also important to recognize when professional guidance is needed. Consult with qualified healthcare providers, such as herbalists, naturopaths, or integrative medicine practitioners, especially if you have chronic health conditions, are taking prescription medications, or are pregnant or breastfeeding. Professional guidance ensures safe and effective use of herbal remedies in conjunction with other treatments.

Continued Exploration and Experimentation

Herbal medicine is a dynamic and evolving field. New research, discoveries, and traditional wisdom continue to enrich our understanding of herbs and their applications. Stay curious and open-minded, and don't be afraid to experiment with new herbs and preparations. Keep a journal of your experiences, noting what works and what doesn't, and use this as a valuable resource for your ongoing herbal practice.

Final Thoughts

Herbal remedies are a gift from nature, offering gentle yet powerful support for our health and well-being. By integrating herbs into our daily lives, we can enhance our vitality, prevent illness, and address a wide range of health concerns naturally. As you embark on this herbal journey, may you find joy, healing, and a deeper connection

Barbara O'Neill Herbal Remedies

to the natural world.

Remember, the path to health and wellness is a lifelong journey. Continue to learn, grow, and thrive, and may the wisdom of the herbs guide you every step of the way.

Thank You

Thank you for embarking on this journey through the world of herbal remedies. May this book serve as a valuable guide and companion, inspiring you to explore, experiment, and embrace the healing power of nature.

Barbara O'Neill Herbal Remedies

Acknowledgments

To all the herbalists, researchers, and traditional healers who have shared their knowledge and wisdom, thank you for your contributions to the field of herbal medicine. Your dedication and passion continue to inspire and guide us.

To the readers, thank you for your interest and commitment to natural health. May your herbal journey be filled with discovery, healing, and well-being.

Resources and Further Reading

For those who wish to delve deeper into the world of herbal medicine, the following resources and recommended readings provide valuable information and insights:

Books

"The Complete Medicinal Herbal" by Penelope Ody

"James Green's book "The Herbal Medicine-Maker's Handbook"

"Encyclopedia of Herbal Medicine" by Andrew Chevallier

Websites

American Herbalists Guild (www.americanherbalistsguild.com)

Herbal Academy (www.theherbalacademy.com)

Mountain Rose Herbs (www.mountainroseherbs.com)

Barbara O'Neill Herbal Remedies

Courses

Herbal Medicine for Everyone by the Herbal Academy

Foundations of Herbalism by Chestnut School of Herbal Medicine

Online Herbal Immersion Program by the Herb Pharm

By exploring these resources, you can continue to expand your knowledge and enjoy a healthy and vital life.

Barbara O'Neill Herbal Remedies

Appendices

The appendices provide additional resources and information to complement your journey into herbal medicine. Here, you'll find detailed references, recipes, and practical tips to enhance your understanding and application of herbal remedies.

Appendix A: Herbal Glossary

A comprehensive glossary of herbal terms and definitions to help you navigate the world of herbal medicine.

Adaptogen: A natural substance that helps the body adapt to stress and promotes overall balance.

Astringent: An herb that tightens tissues and reduces secretions.

Carminative: An herb that helps relieve gas and bloating in the digestive tract.

Decoction: A method of extracting the medicinal properties of herbs by simmering them in water.

Infusion: A method of preparing herbal teas by steeping herbs in hot water.

Poultice: A soft, moist mass of herbs applied to the skin to reduce inflammation or draw out infections.

Barbara O'Neill Herbal Remedies

Tincture: A concentrated liquid extract of herbs made by soaking them in alcohol or glycerin.

Appendix B: Herb-Drug Interactions

Important information on potential interactions between herbs and pharmaceuticals.

St. John's Wort (Hypericum perforatum): Can interact with antidepressants, birth control pills, and blood thinners, reducing their effectiveness.

Ginkgo Biloba: When combined with blood thinners like warfarin, it may make bleeding more likely.

Garlic (Allium sativum): Can enhance the effects of anticoagulant medications, increasing the risk of bleeding.

Echinacea (Echinacea purpurea): May interact with immunosuppressant drugs, potentially reducing their effectiveness.

Prior to taking prescription drugs along with natural therapies, always get medical advice.

Barbara O'Neill Herbal Remedies

Appendix C: Herbal Recipes

A collection of recipes for making your own herbal preparations at home.

Basic Herbal Infusion

One or two tablespoons of fresh herbs, or one or two teaspoons of dried herbs

1 cup of boiling water

Pour boiling water over the herbs, cover, and steep for 10-15 minutes. Strain and enjoy.

Herbal Tincture

1 part dried herbs or 2 parts fresh herbs

5 parts alcohol (vodka or brandy)

Place herbs in a glass jar and cover with alcohol. Seal tightly and store in a cool, dark place for 4-6 weeks, shaking daily. Strain and bottle the tincture.

Herbal Salve

1 cup infused herbal oil (e.g., calendula or comfrey)

1/4 cup beeswax

Melt beeswax in a double boiler and add the herbal oil. Stir until

Barbara O'Neill Herbal Remedies

combined, then pour into containers and allow to cool and solidify.

Appendix D: Herb Growing Calendar

A seasonal guide to planting, growing, and harvesting herbs.

Spring

Plant seeds of basil, dill, and parsley indoors.

Transplant seedlings of rosemary, thyme, and oregano outdoors after the last frost.

Summer

Harvest herbs like mint, cilantro, and basil regularly to encourage growth.

Dry or freeze herbs for later use.

Autumn

Plant garlic cloves for harvest next summer.

Harvest and dry perennial herbs like sage, rosemary, and thyme.

Winter

Grow herbs like chives, parsley, and basil indoors in pots.

Make plans for your garden's upcoming growth season.

Barbara O'Neill Herbal Remedies

Appendix E: Resources and References

A curated list of books, websites, and organizations for further exploration of herbal medicine.

Books

"The Complete Medicinal Herbal" by Penelope Ody

James Green's book "The Herbal Medicine-Maker's Handbook"

"Encyclopedia of Herbal Medicine" by Andrew Chevallier

Websites

American Herbalists Guild: www.americanherbalistsguild.com

Herbal Academy: www.theherbalacademy.com

Mountain Rose Herbs: www.mountainroseherbs.com

Organizations

American Botanical Council: Promotes the responsible use of herbal medicine.

National Institute of Medical Herbalists: Professional organization for herbal practitioners.

United Plant Savers: Focuses on the conservation of at-risk medicinal plants.

Barbara O'Neill Herbal Remedies

Appendix F: Herbal Safety Guidelines

Essential tips for using herbs safely and effectively.

Start Slowly: Introduce new herbs one at a time to monitor your body's response.

Dosage: Follow recommended dosages and consult with a healthcare professional for personalized advice.

Quality: Use high-quality, organic herbs to avoid contaminants and ensure potency.

Allergies: Be aware of potential allergies and sensitivities. In the event that you have negative responses, stop using.

Pregnancy and Breastfeeding: Some herbs are not safe during pregnancy or breastfeeding. Consult a medical professional before to use.

These appendices serve as a valuable resource, providing detailed information and practical tips to support your herbal practice. Whether you are a beginner or an experienced herbalist, these additional insights and tools will enhance your understanding and application of herbal remedies.

www.ingramcontent.com/pod-product-compliance
Lightning Source LLC
Chambersburg PA
CBHW050802250726

48653CB00006B/2038